Lollipops, Chocolate, Donuts, or Cake?

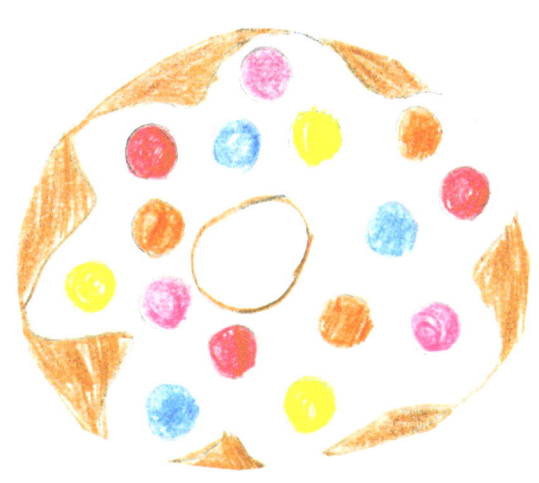

Dr. Daniel Materna

Description

"Lollipops, Chocolate, Donuts or Cake? Eating is fun, but what you don't know is the trouble it can make," says Dr. Daniel Materna's son Ryan who, with his sister Joslyn, created the colored illustrations for this book. The book poetically tells the story in a whimsical fashion about the pleasures and perplexing problems eating can entail. In the end, the poem highlights a specific recipe to solve eating troubles that both children and adults can savor. The book is fun, entertaining, and surprisingly effective in highlighting solutions to even the most serious of eating disorders.

The Author

Dr. Daniel Materna is a clinical psychologist who operates a private practice with his wife "Dr. Jill" in Hermitage, PA. "Dr. Dan" has evaluated many severely obese patients preparing for gastric bypass surgeries and has worked to help others lessen addictions to emotional eating habits. Lollipops, Chocolate, Donuts, or Cake? summarizes the lessons he has learned in helping people overcome uncontrolled relationships with food.

Copies of the book can be ordered through:
Materna Psychological Services, P.C.
701 N. Hermitage Rd., Suite 9
Hermitage, PA 16148
724-346-4510

Available on Amazon.com and other retailers

Dedication

This book is dedicated to all those who have mistakenly sought comfort, love, and nurturance through food.

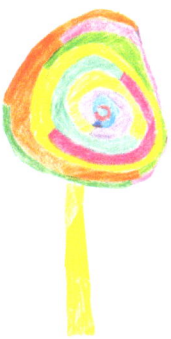

Acknowledgement

Thanks to Joslyn and Ryan for investing their creative energies into the book's illustrations and the thoughtful ways they depict the poem's content and meanings. Also, thanks to local editor Judith McConville. Her ability to see the good or potential in projects helps get writing tasks done with less hesitation.

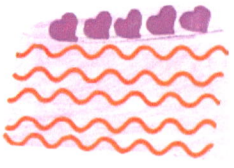

Lollipops, Chocolate, Donuts, or Cake?

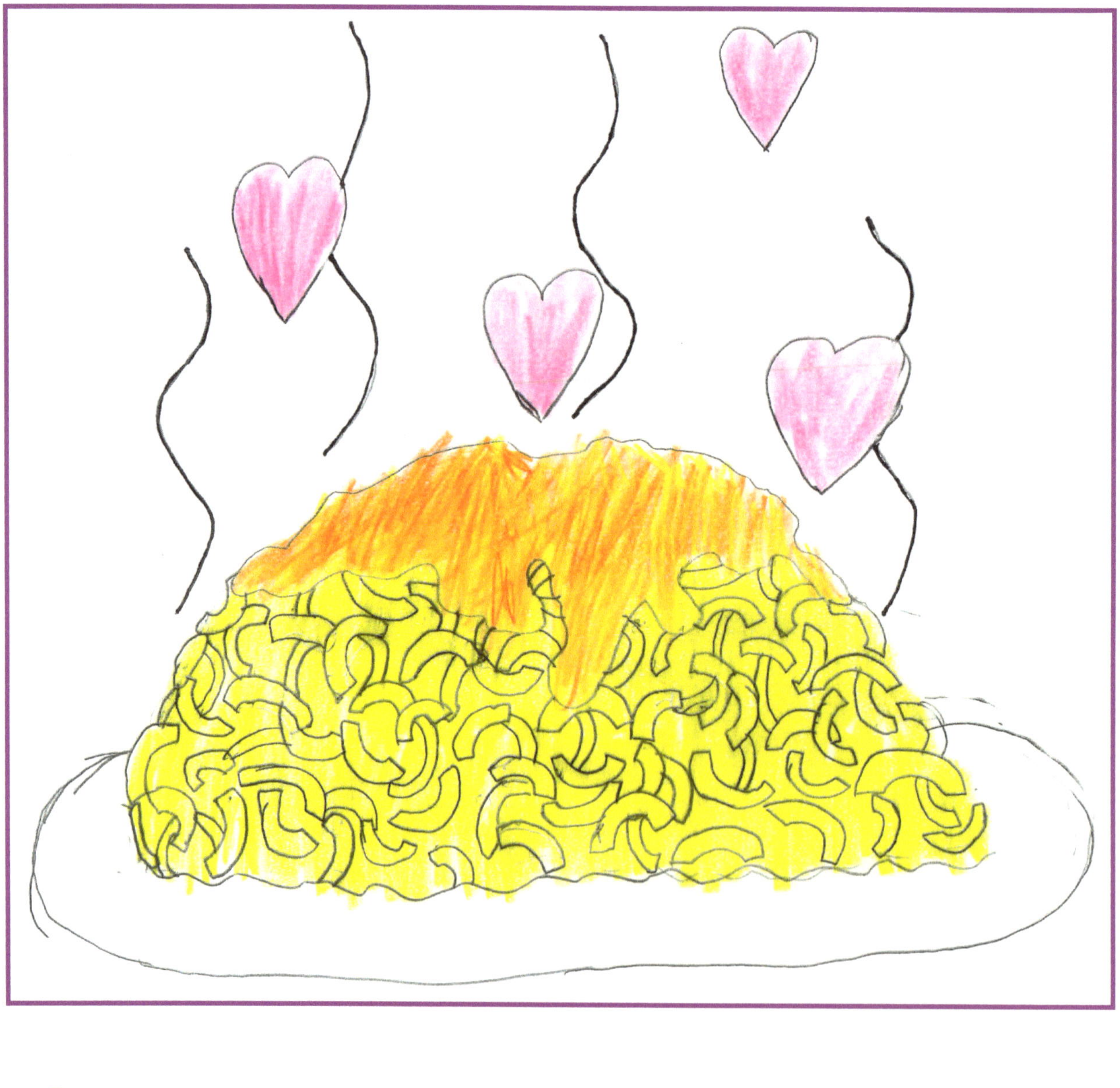

Lollipops, Chocolate, Donuts or Cake?
How do you like yours - fried, battered or baked?
Macaroni and cheese tastes good,
Warms my tummy - so divine!
And when baked by grandma,
The pasta, cheese, and love are really, really, fine.
Lollipops, Chocolate, Donuts or Cake?

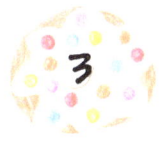

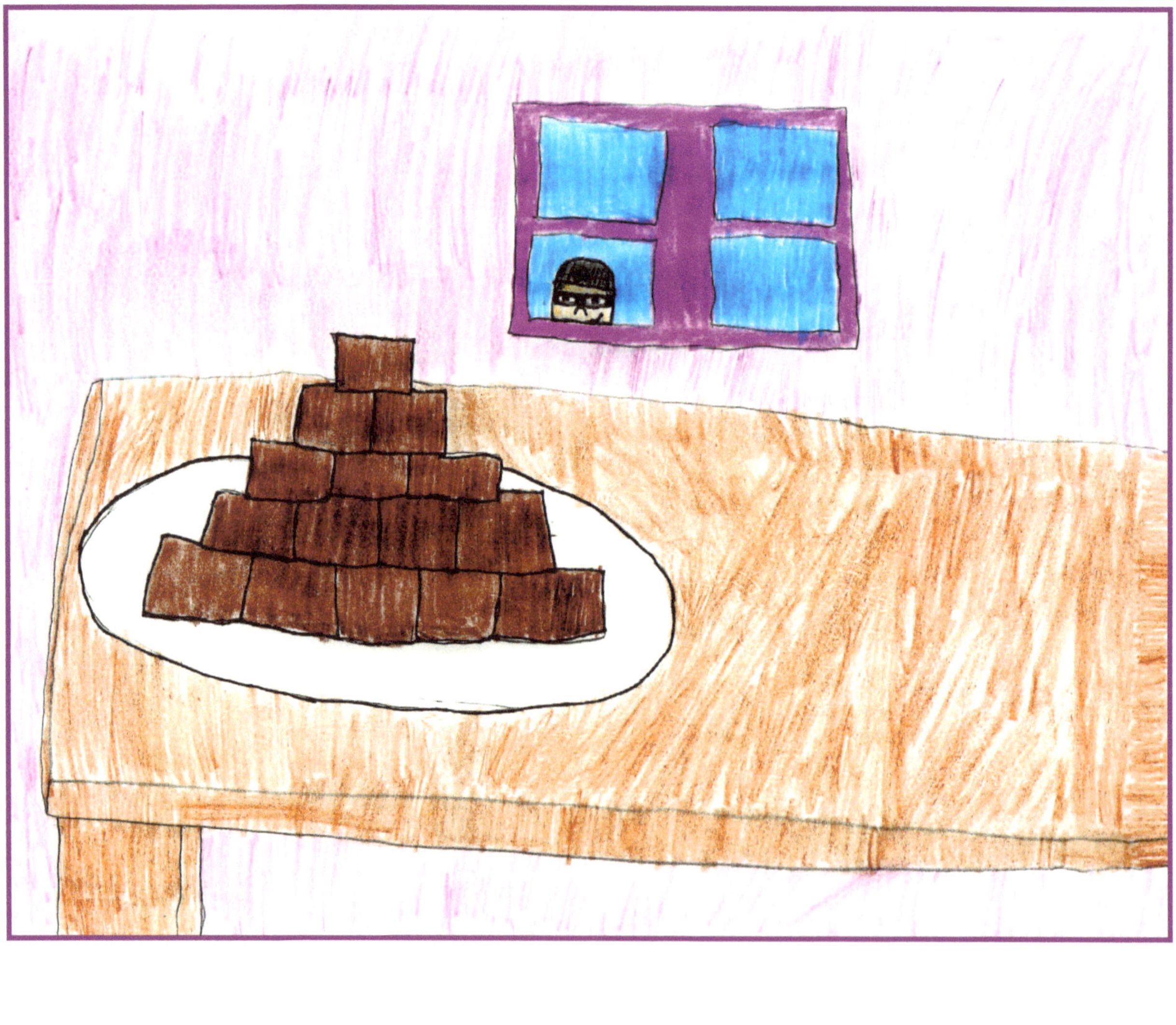

And don't try and steal my chocolates,
Don't you even think twice.
I <u>need</u> my treats.
'Cause they taste oh so nice!
Lollipops, Chocolate, Donuts or Cake?

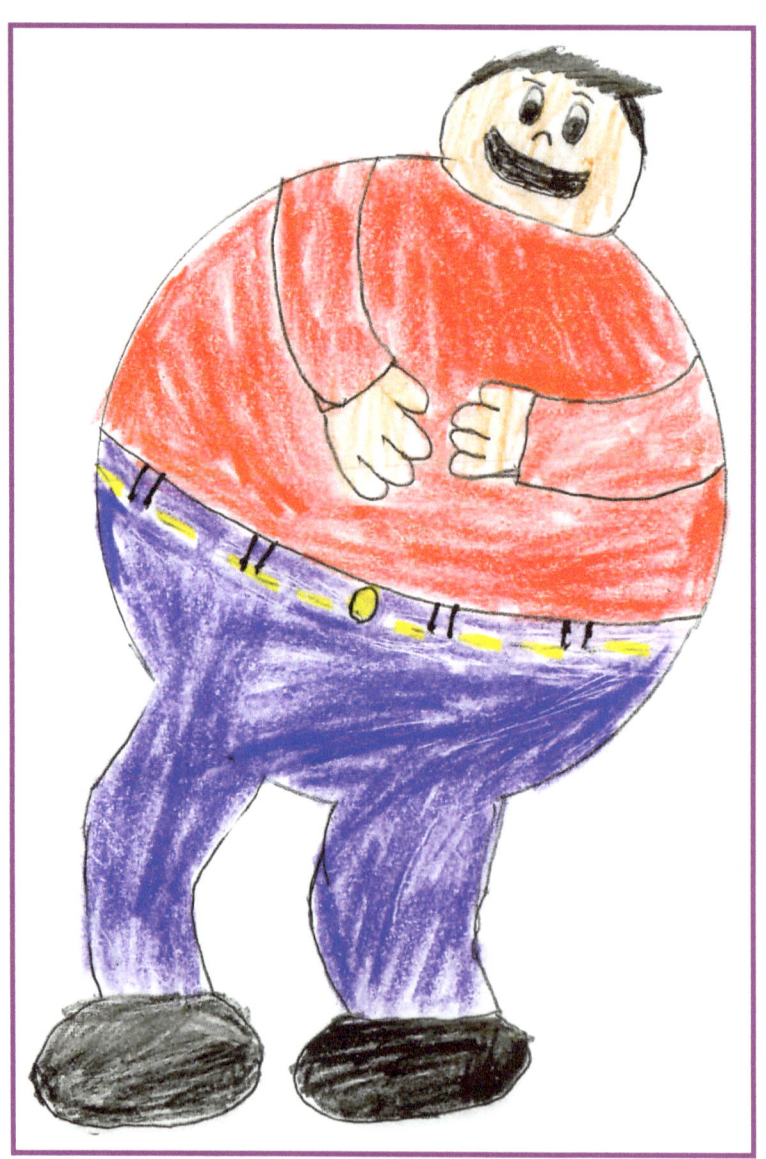

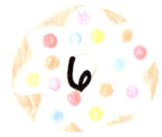

But the warmth in my stomach,
And sweet taste on my tongue,
Want me to ignore my expanding waistline.
And it's only just begun...
Lollipops, Chocolate, Donuts or Cake?

GUMMY
COOKIE
CANDY
CHOCOLATE

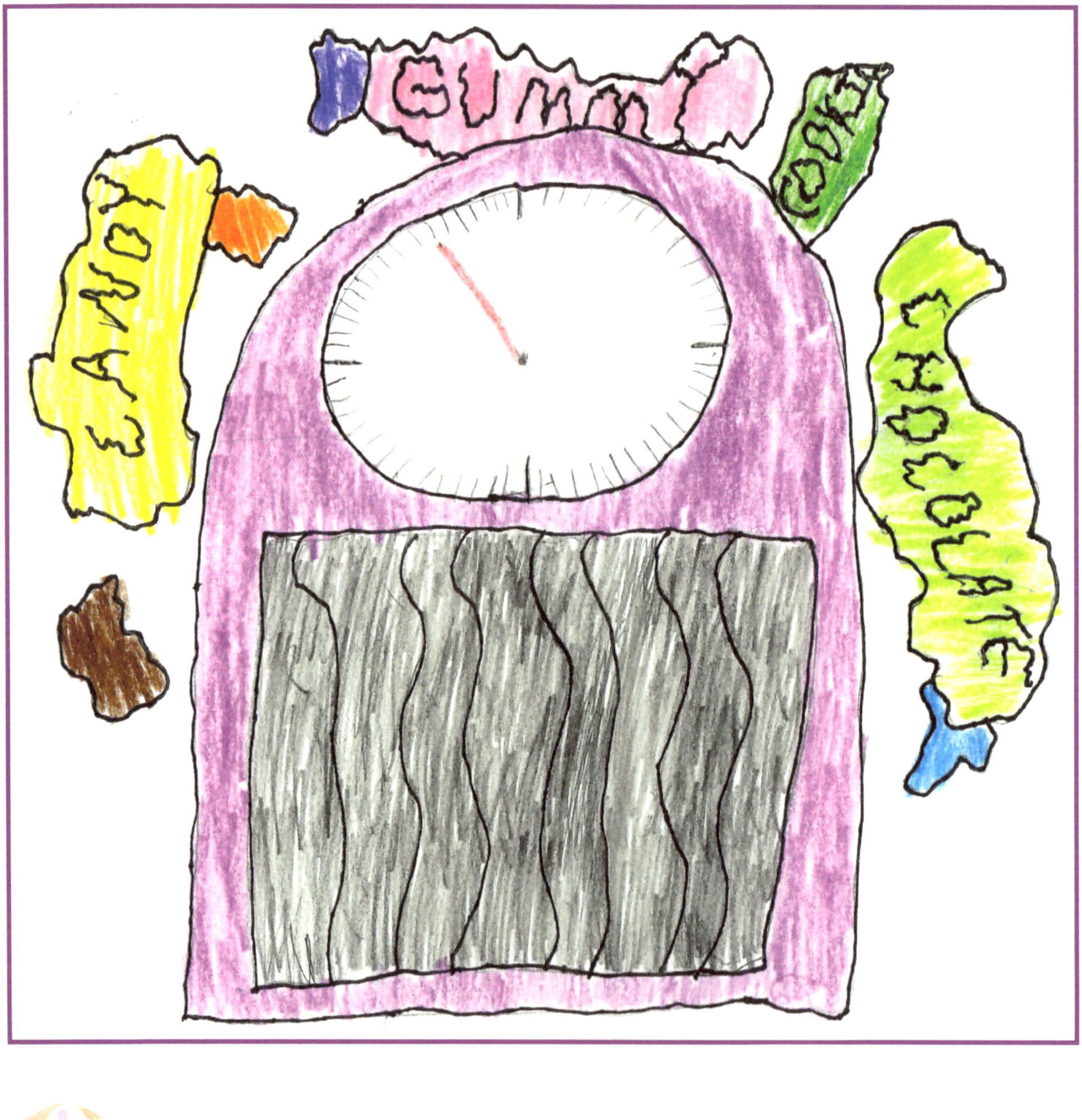

You see, those rising numbers on my scale,
And extra inches around my waist,
Trigger some concern,
To which I do not wait.
So, I pop another chocolate,
And avoid the mirror, just in case!
Lollipops, Chocolate, Donuts or Cake?

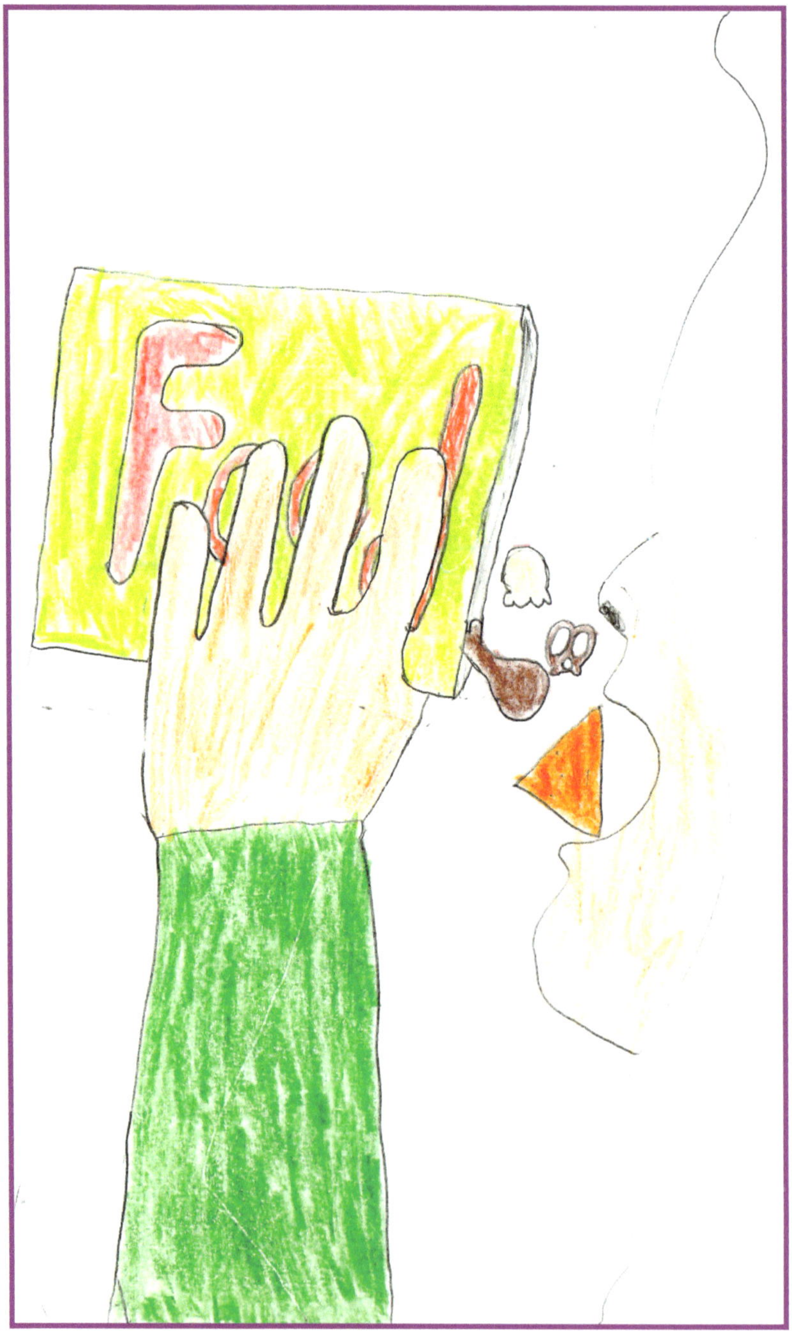

10

Now some people, I have heard,
Have eating problems of different sorts;
Some stuff too much in,

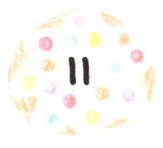

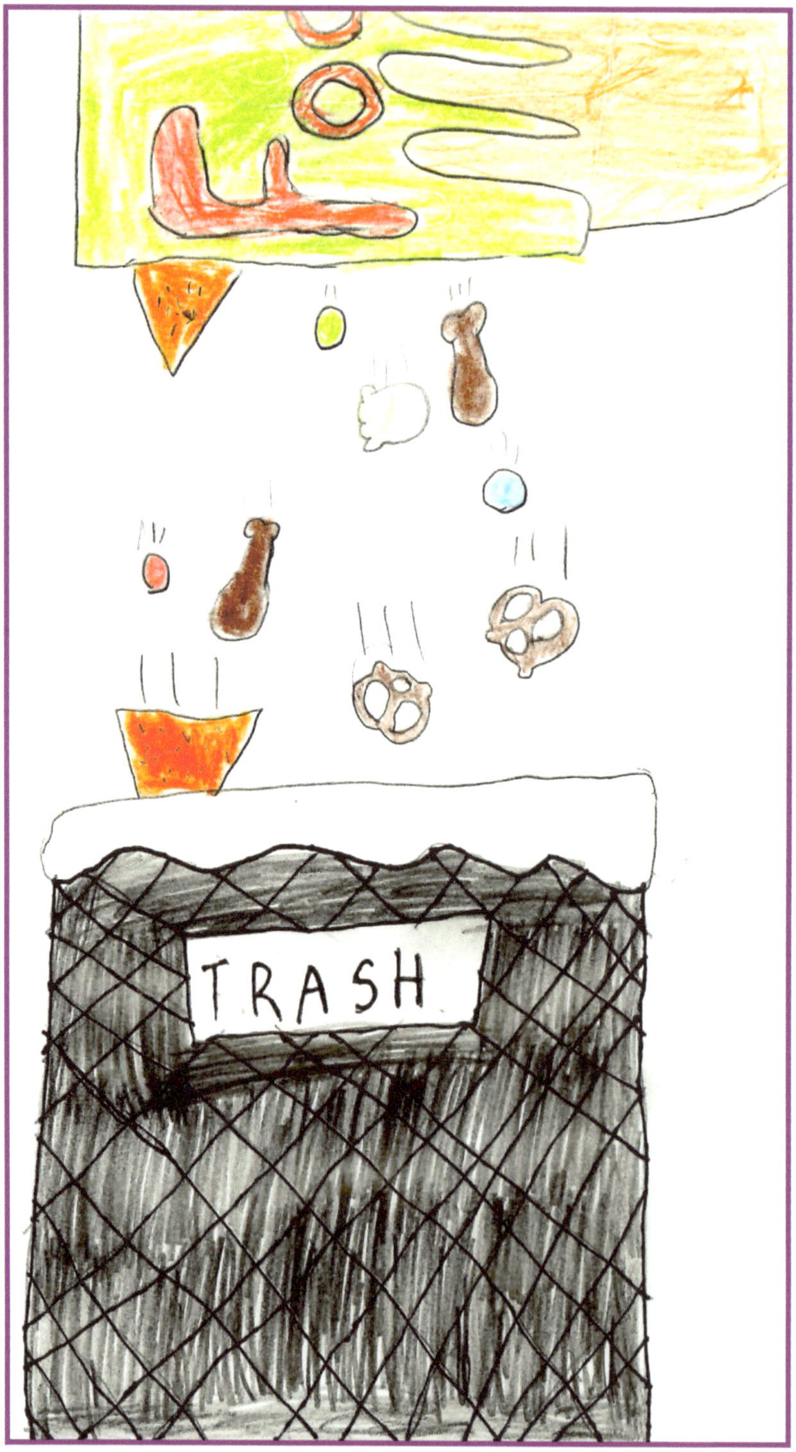

While others want to throw it all back out.

A few refuse attempts to control them,

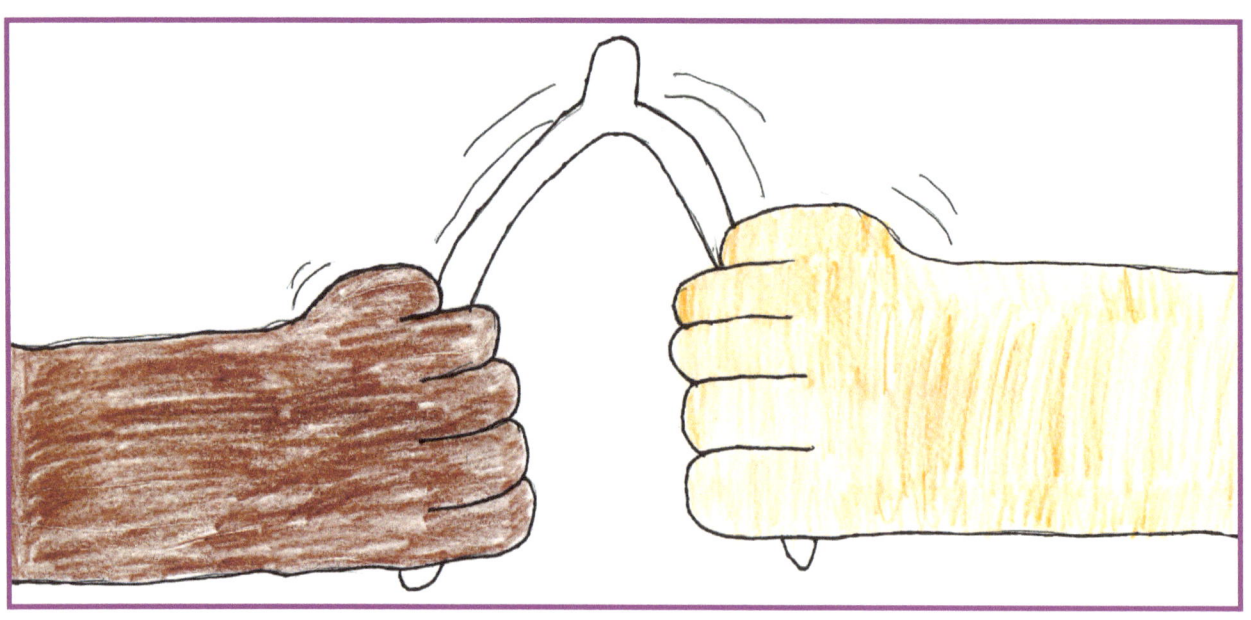

They'll continue till just skin and bones.
But what's the battle about?
Why do we hide it all alone?
Lollipops, Chocolate, Donuts or Cake?

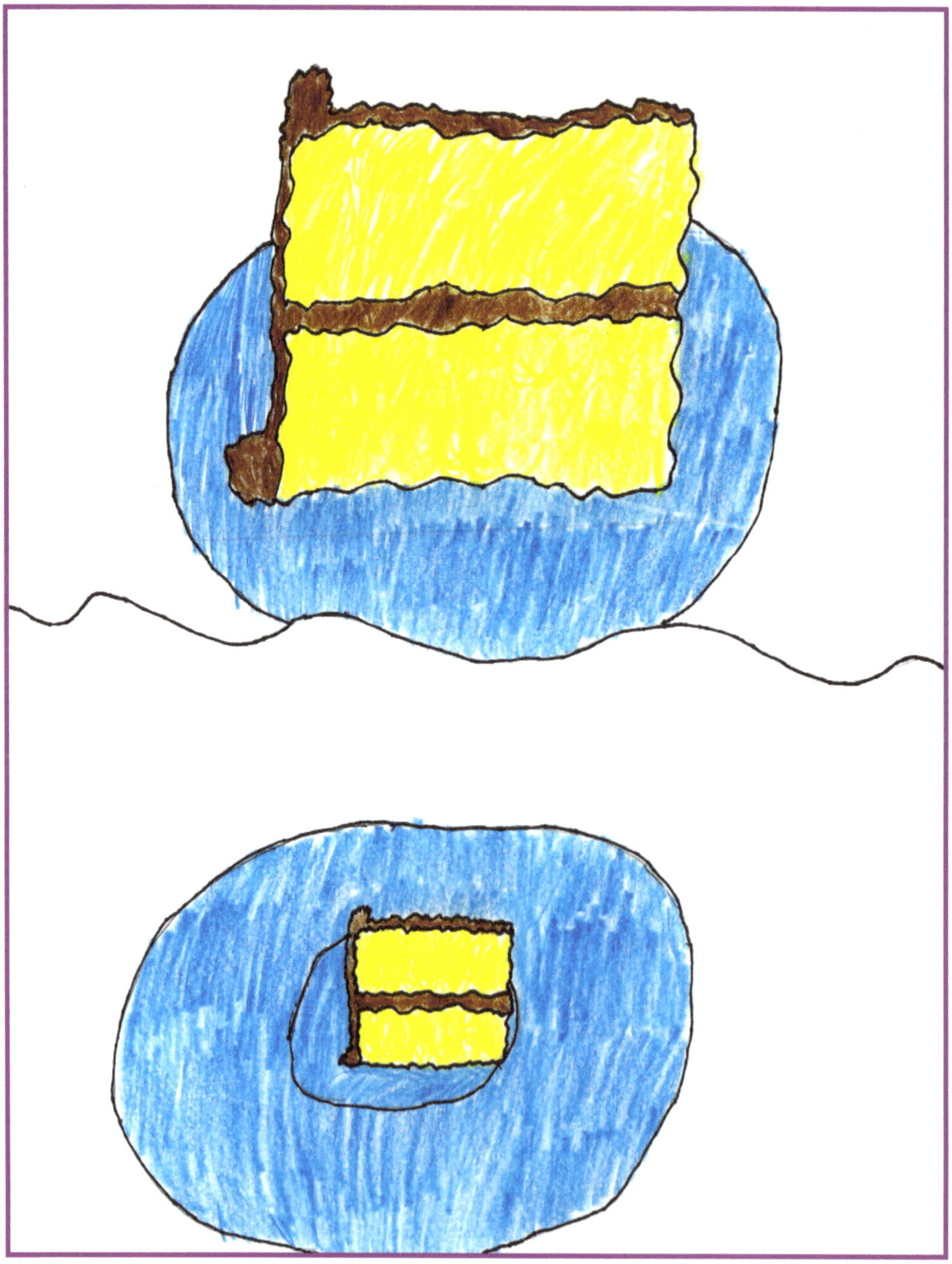

Thus, some love foods too much,
And some want less than a little.
What is it about food?
Are we really that fickle?
Lollipops, Chocolate, Donuts or Cake?

18

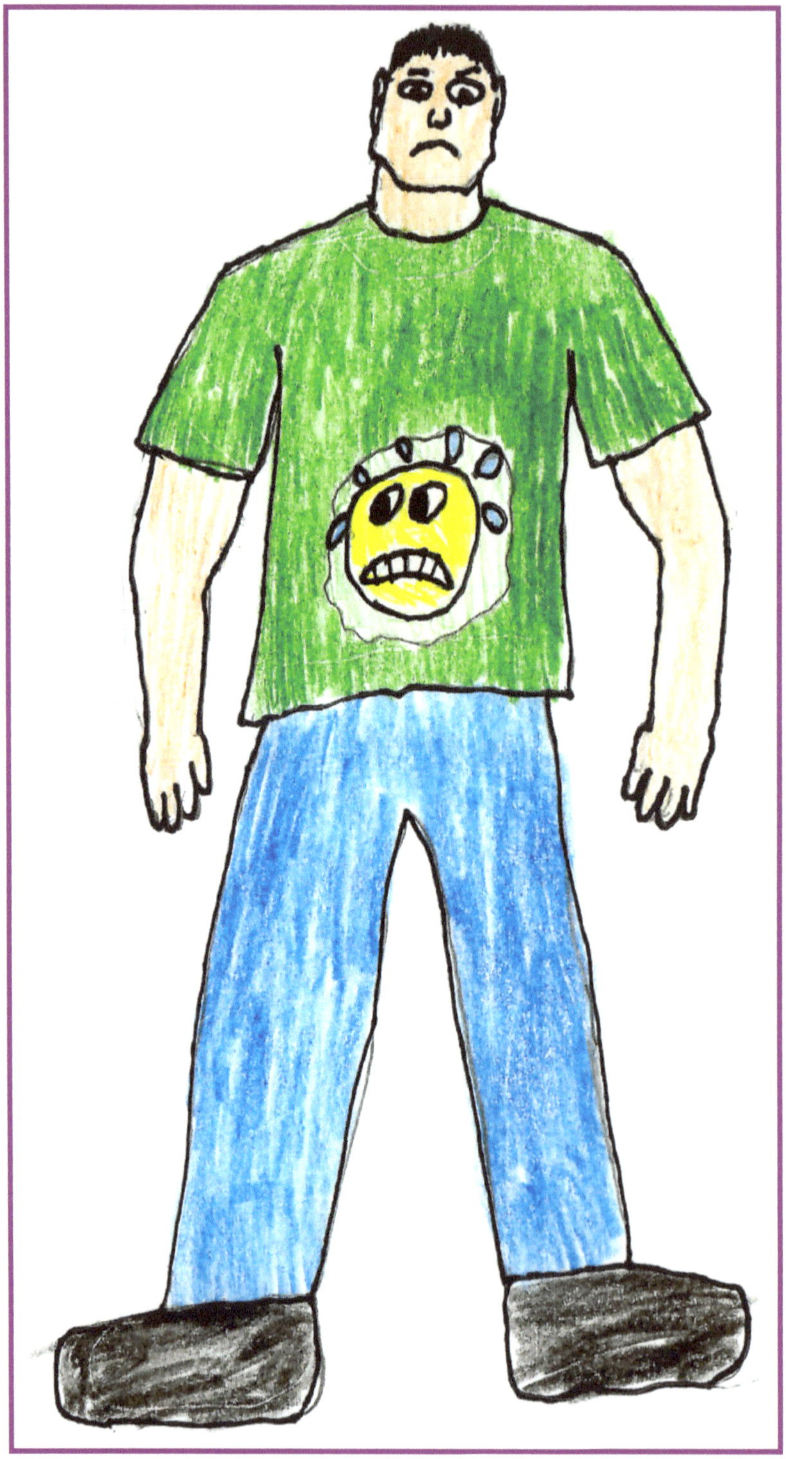

But it's hard to have just one,
And to eat in moderation,
If your stomach feels all stirred up,
Or if your mind is constantly searching.

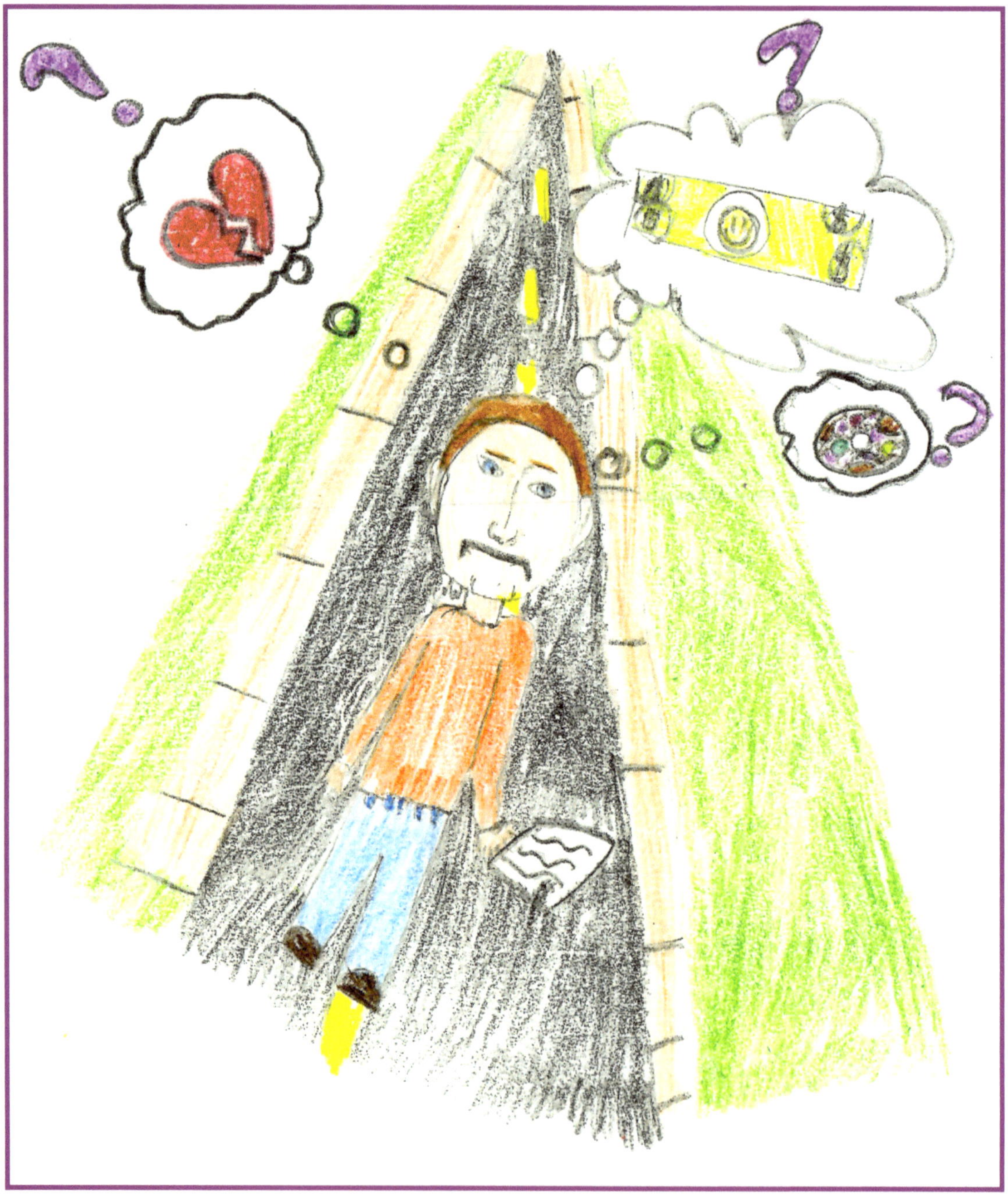

You see that empty feeling deep inside,
Or extra thoughts that you've been having,
Might indicate a different kind of problem –
Maybe one that you're denying.
Lollipops, Chocolate, Donuts or Cake?

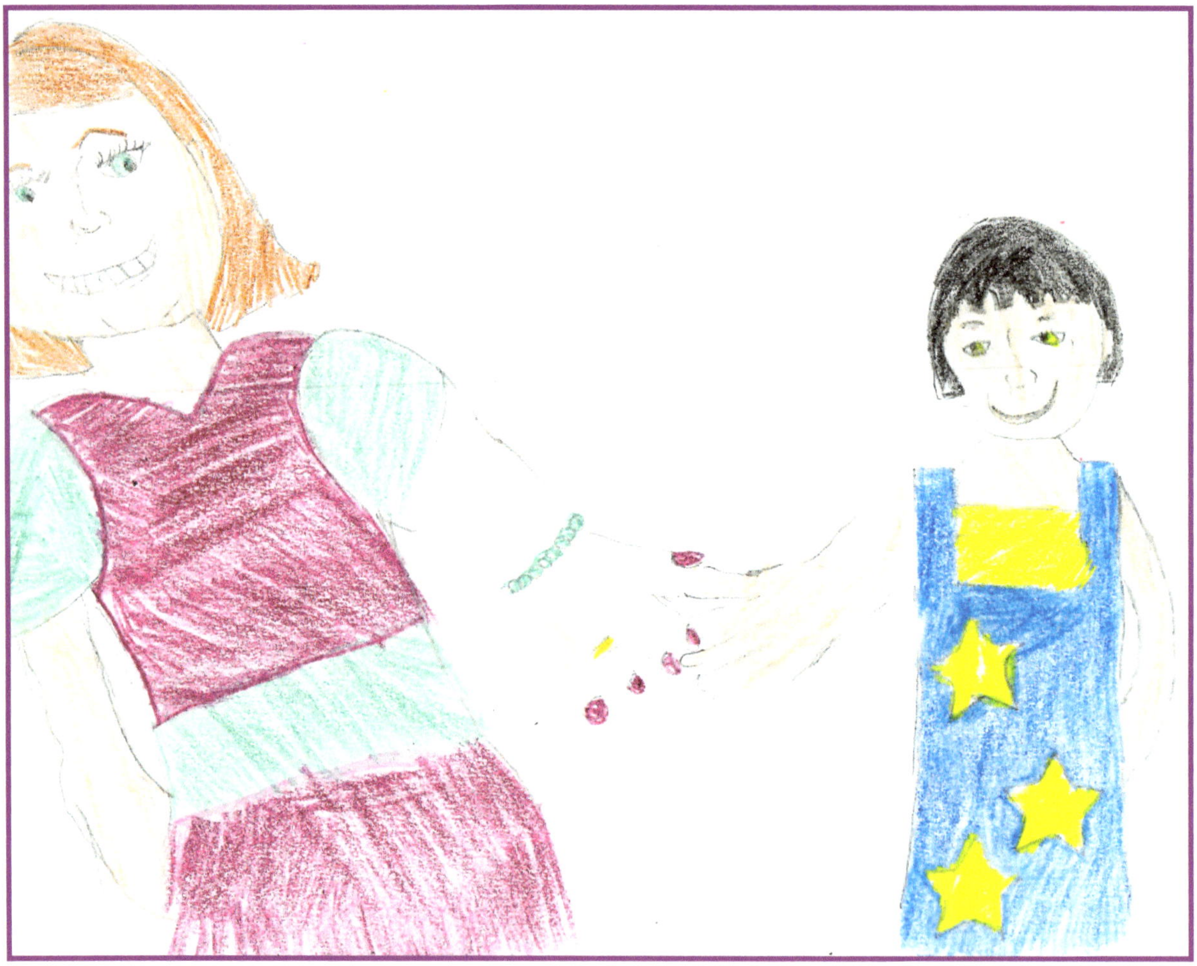

Now, if you get your love from food,
Or if you claim your independence through its rejection;
It might be you that you are fooling,
A lack of safe and secure love may be the problem.
Lollipops, Chocolate, Donuts or Cake?

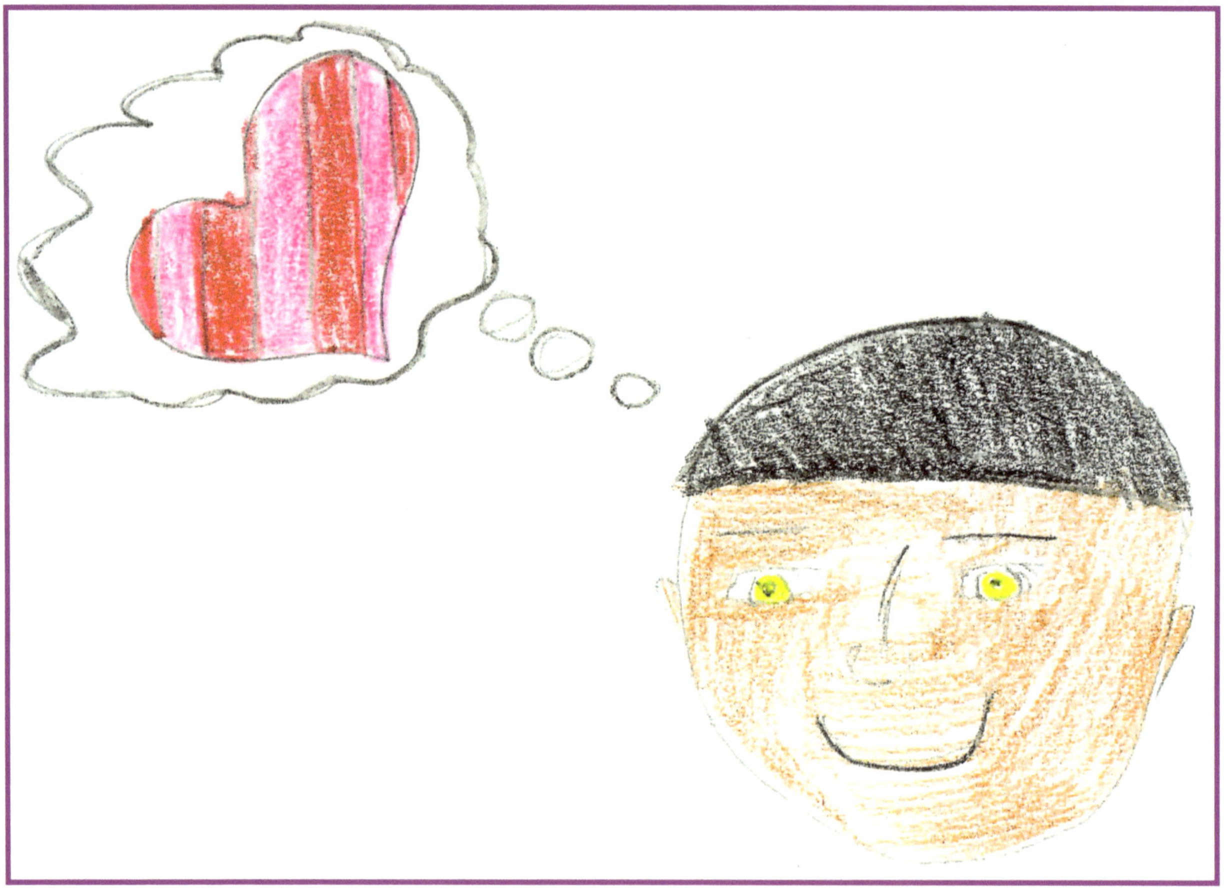

So take a moment to reflect,
What your needs are all about.
If it's another's love that you are craving,
If it's safe and secure love that you are
really searching out.
Stay away from food for this purpose,
And don't give it further doubt.
Lollipops, Chocolate, Donuts or Cake?

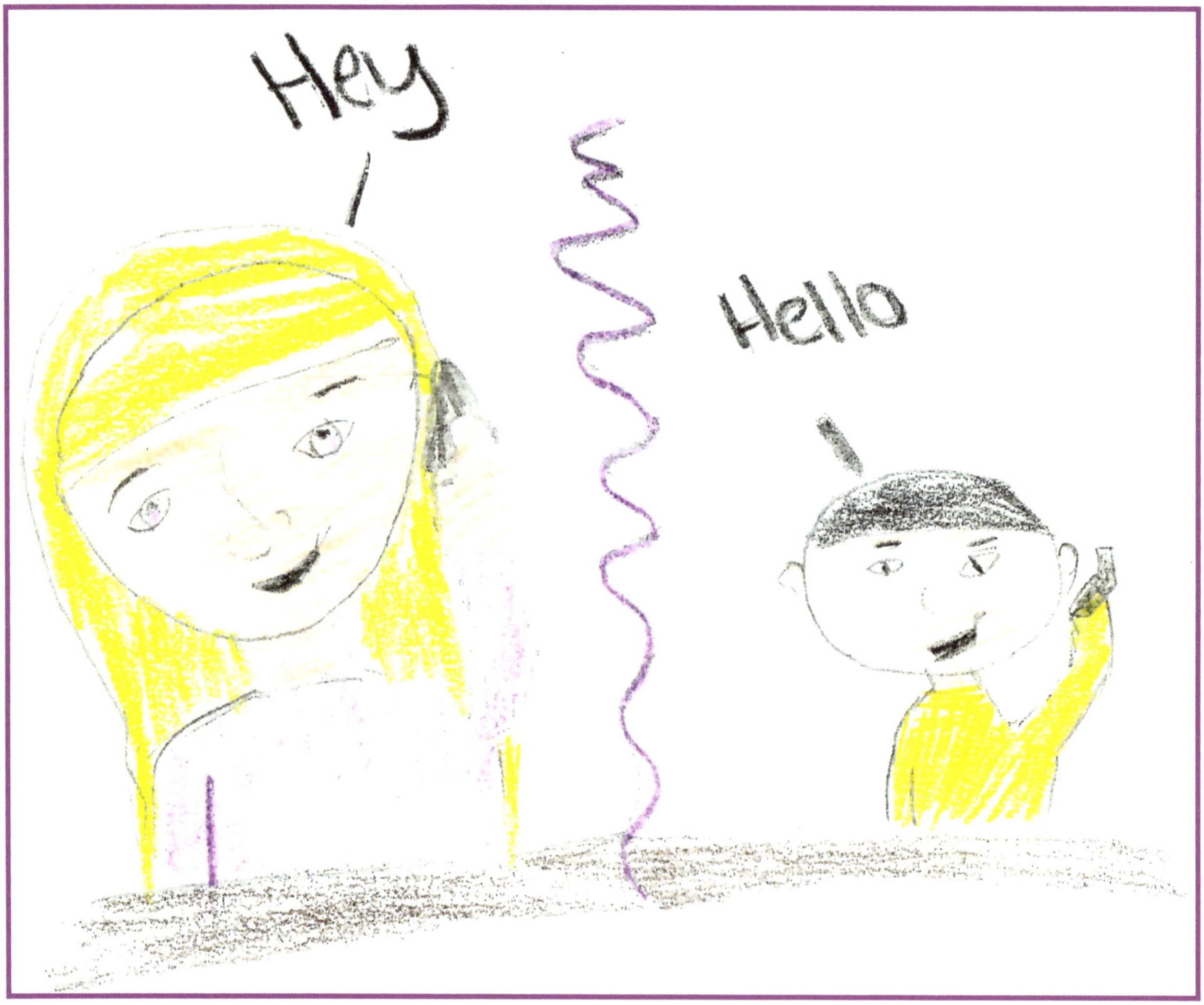

Instead, ask someone to come over;
Or ask them to meet you out.

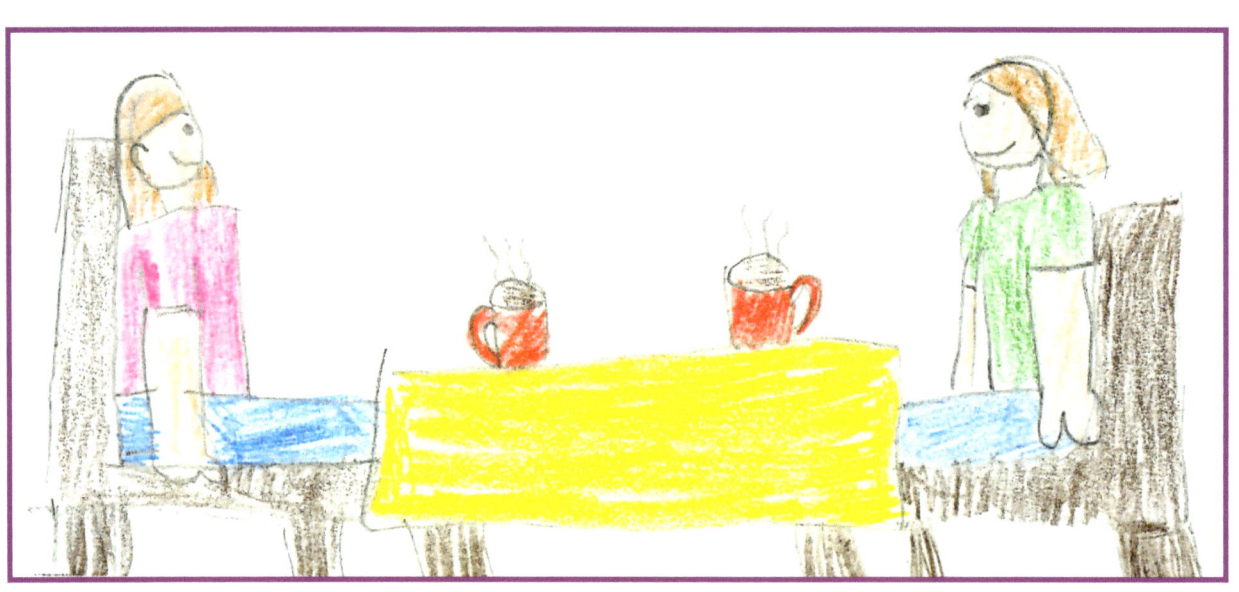

Tell them what you need,
Tell them what you are all about.
But be sure to return the favor,

Are You having fun?
I'm having fun!
Me too

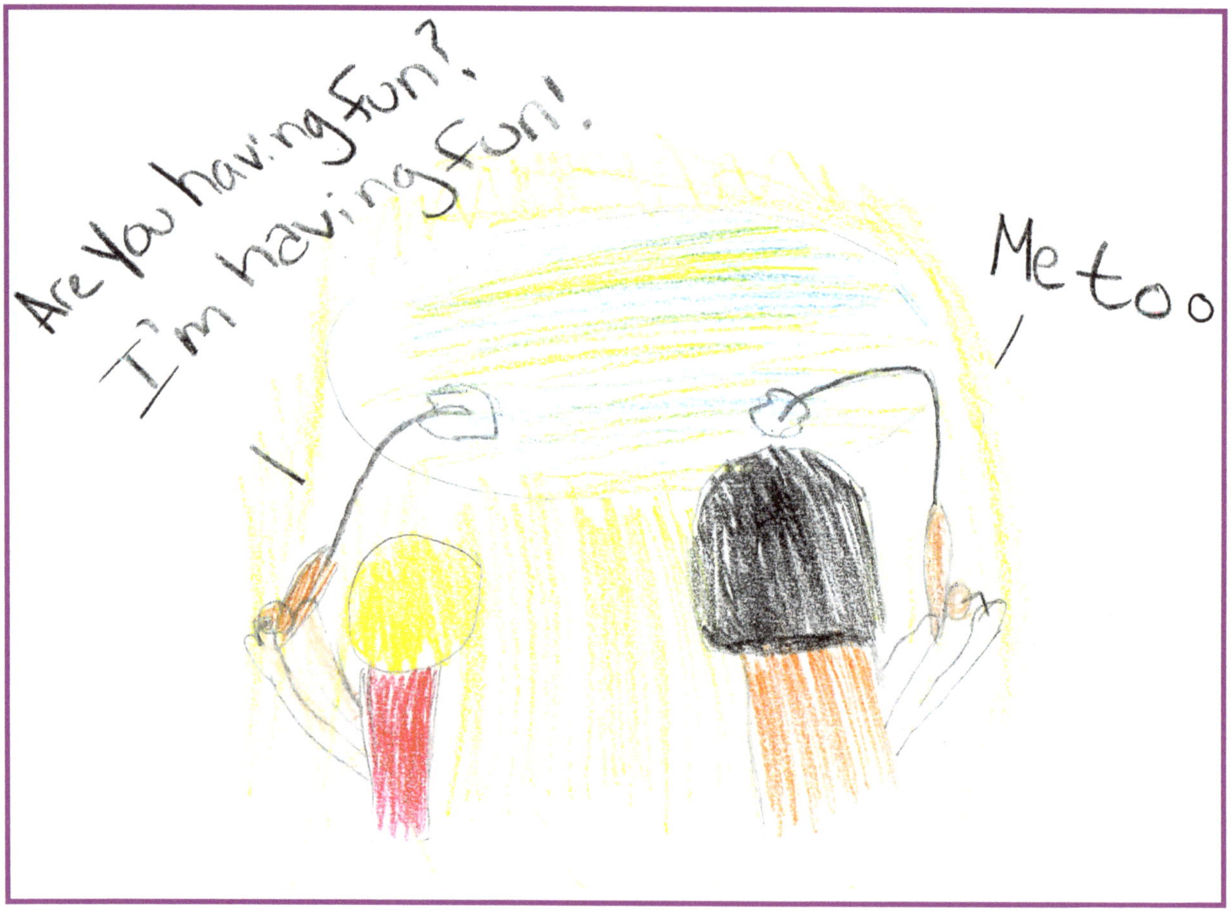

Ask your friends of their needs too.

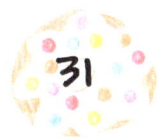

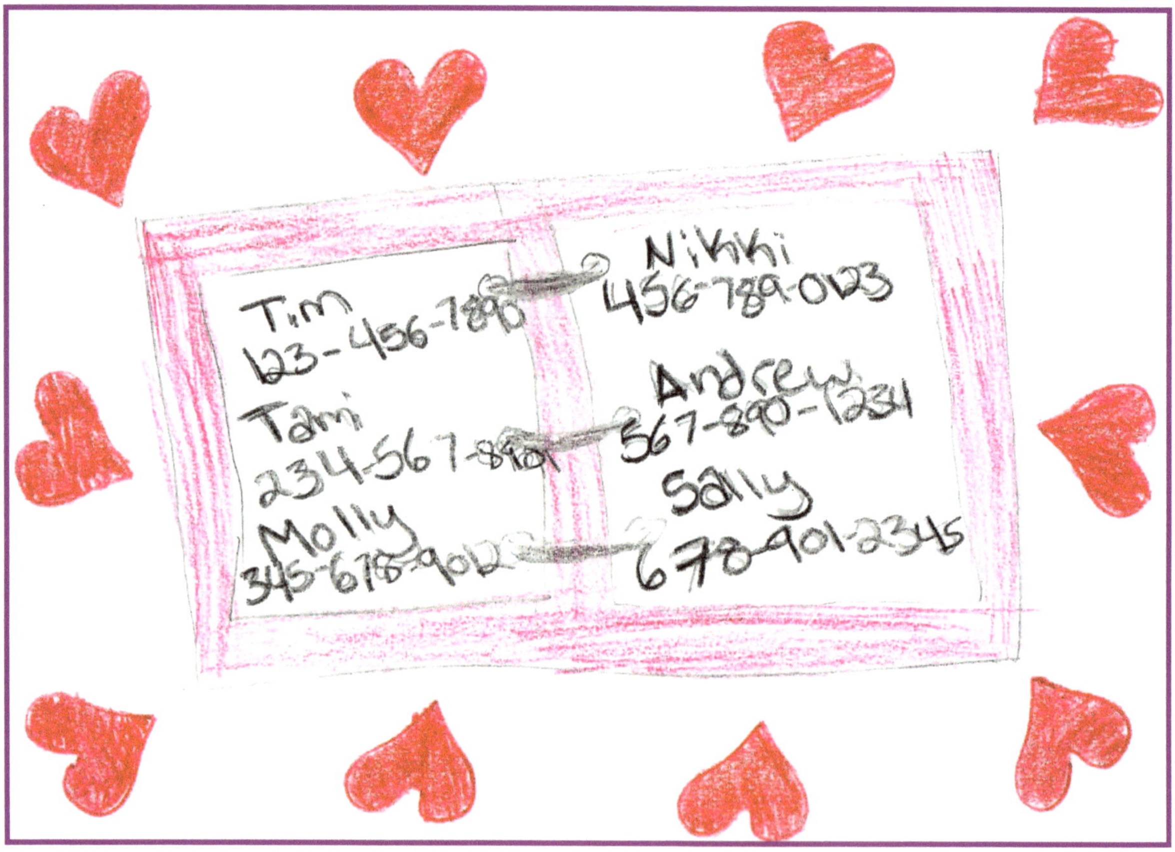

Tim
123-456-7890
Tami
234-567-8901
Molly
345-678-9012

Nikki
456-789-0123
Andrew
567-890-1234
Sally
678-901-2345

You see love must come from people,
And it is something you must pursue!
Lollipops, Chocolate, Donuts or Cake?

www.ingramcontent.com/pod-product-compliance
Lightning Source LLC
Chambersburg PA
CBHW041531280526
45792CB00004B/1461